QUINOA

The Nutritional Powerhouse and Versatile Grain for Healthy Living (2023 Guide for Beginners)

Sophia Bates

Understanding Quinoa Varieties

Quinoas are most usually seen in white/golden, red, and black varieties.

In terms of flavour, all quinoa has a nutty flavour that is somewhat bitter. The tastes, however, are faint and unlikely to impact the overall flavour of a meal. According to some cooks, white quinoa is the mildest and least crunchy, while black quinoa has the earthiest flavour and is the chewiest. The red is somewhere in the middle.

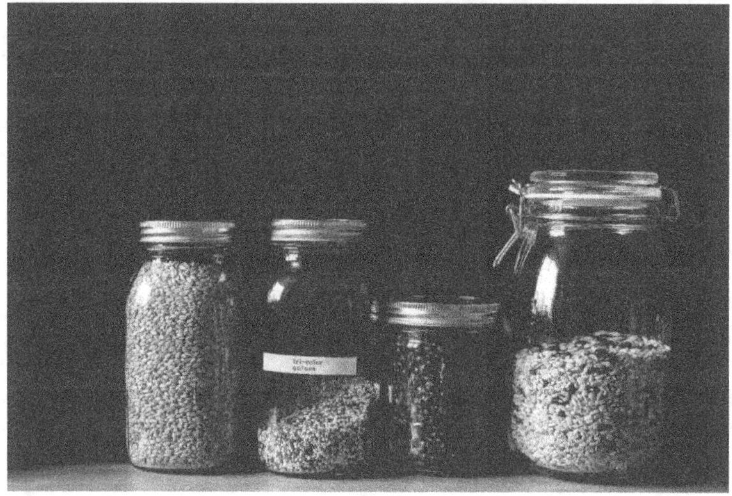

All forms of quinoa, whether red, black, or white, have the same basic advantages of being low in calories and rich in protein, and they have essentially comparable nutritional content. Choosing the proper quinoa to utilize may be as simple as deciding on the colour that would be most attractive for the dish. Red quinoa, for example, looks great in a salad with edamame, black beans, maize, and red cabbage, but black quinoa goes well with fresh salad leaves, cherry tomatoes, cashews, and red pomegranate seeds.

How to Purchase and Store Quinoa

Buy quinoa packages with no rips or holes, since moisture might harm their freshness. Once you've settled on your preferred brand, you may purchase it in bulk to save money.

Choose pre-washed quinoa since it is much simpler to deal with and safer to cook with. Raw quinoa grains are naturally covered with a bitter-tasting chemical component known as saponins, which may be somewhat poisonous. Even if you purchased pre-washed quinoa, it is best to rinse it under running water before cooking.

After opening the package, place the quinoa in an airtight container and keep it dry for 2-3 years on a kitchen shelf or in the refrigerator. However, the older the grains, the longer they will take to cook.

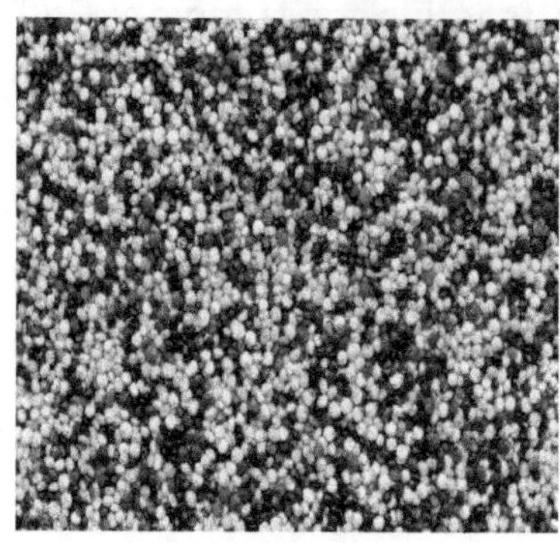 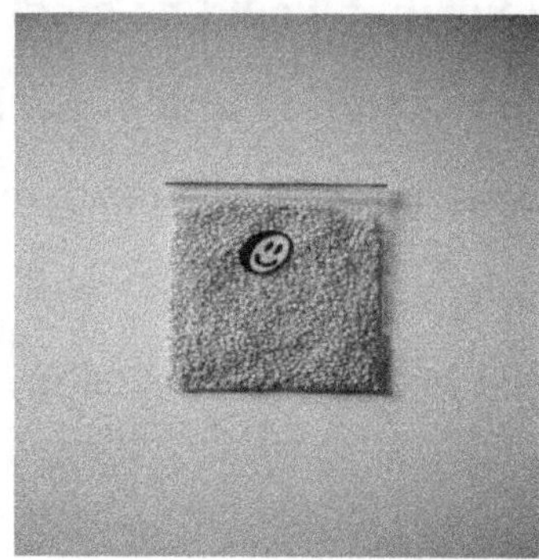

How to Cook Quinoa

The same fundamental methods are used to prepare all forms of quinoa.

To begin, always rinse your quinoa. This is true even if you purchased pre-washed quinoa since quinoa has a natural coating called saponin, which may cause it to taste bitter or soapy and can be mildly poisonous. Rinse the quinoa in a fine-mesh sieve or colander under running water for approximately a minute or two. Shake off any excess water after a few vigorous rubs.

Next, depending on how much quinoa you're making, add it to a small to a medium-sized pot. A cup of uncooked dry quinoa yields 3 cups of cooked quinoa, so don't overload the pot. To cook the quinoa, the quinoa-to-liquid ratio should be roughly 1:2, but the black type may need a bit more. Water is the usual method, but chicken or vegetable broth, or possibly a dab of miso paste, adds a more powerful taste.

Bring the liquid to a boil over high heat, then lower it to medium heat and continue to simmer for another 15 minutes, or until most of the liquid has been absorbed. Some recipes call for covering the pot while the quinoa cooks. I found that not covering the liquid allows it to drain quickly while maintaining its texture. When you notice little spirals or a 'tail' emerge from the quinoa, it's done.

Remove the saucepan from the heat and cover it with a lid. Allow it to rest in the steam for around 10-15 minutes to continue cooking. After that, fluff it with a fork. Season with a healthy quantity of salt, pepper, and spices according to taste.

Another option for cooking the quinoa is to toast it beforehand. In the saucepan, dry out the rinsed quinoa over medium heat. Add a teaspoon of cooking oil after most of the liquid has evaporated. Cook the quinoa until it becomes brown and begins to pop, approximately 10-15 minutes. To avoid burning, keep an eye on the quinoa and stir it constantly. When it's beautifully browned, pour in the liquid and simmer according to the directions above. The extra step of toasting will improve the overall taste of the meal.

A rice cooker is another simple technique of preparation.

Add the ingredients to the cooker, 1 part quinoa to 2 parts liquid. Turn it on according to the manufacturer's directions, and you'll have cooked quinoa in no time.

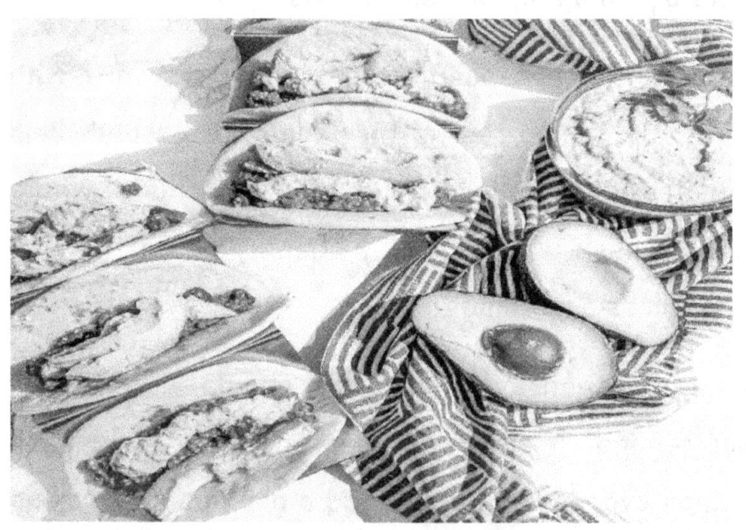

Recipes for Breakfast

Strawberry and Banana Breakfast Quinoa

Servings: 2

Ingredients

1 cup of water

½ cup cooked quinoa

a tsp vanilla extract

½ teaspoon ground cinnamon

1 ½ cup milk

1 sliced small banana

½ cup diced strawberries

2 tbsp. almonds, sliced

2 tbsp shredded unsweetened coconut

Preparation

6. Combine the quinoa and water in a medium pot. Bring the water to a boil over high heat before reducing it to a low setting. Allow the quinoa to continue cooking for approximately 15 minutes, or until all of the liquid has been absorbed. Remove from the heat and place a lid on top. Allow it to settle for 5 minutes. Toss the quinoa with a fork after adding the vanilla and cinnamon.

7. Divide the quinoa evenly between two dishes. Fill each dish with equal parts milk and top with banana slices, strawberries, almonds, and shredded coconut.

8. Serve right away.

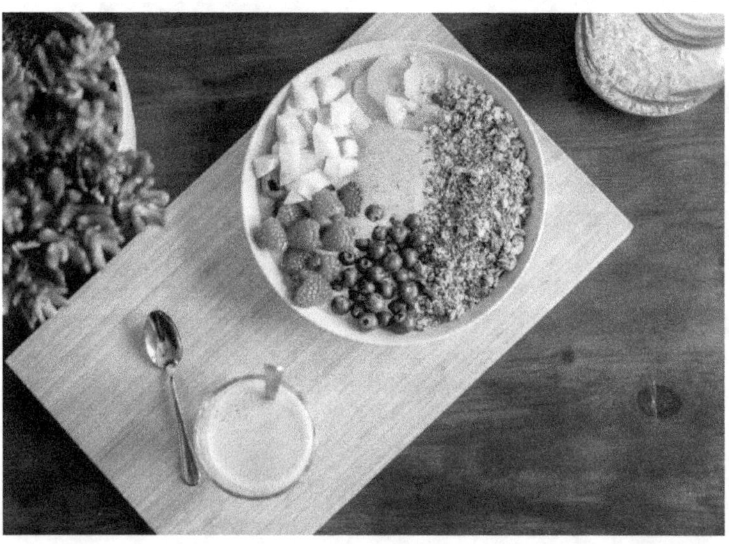

Nutritional Information (301 g per serving)

- Calories 470
- Fats 24 g
- Carbs 54 g
- Protein 15 g
- Sodium 88 mg

Quinoa with Coconut and Cherry Compote

Servings: 4

Ingredients

1 cup of quinoa 1 cup of almond milk

1 can (16 oz.) light coconut milk

1 pound pitted frozen cherries

2 teaspoons water

a pinch of salt

1 teaspoon maple syrup

½ cup coarsely chopped almonds

½ cup shredded unsweetened coconut

Preparation

1. Cook the quinoa in the almond milk in a medium saucepan over medium heat until all of the liquid is absorbed. Next, gently pour in the coconut milk, stirring frequently, until most of the liquid has been absorbed. Keep some coconut milk on the side to keep it creamy and moist. Set aside and cover with a lid.

2. Cook the cherries, water, and a pinch of salt in a small saucepan over low or medium-low heat for approximately 10-15 minutes, to enable the cherries to release their juices. Once the sauce has thickened, add the maple syrup and heat for 2 minutes more. Take the pan off the heat.

3. To assemble, place quinoa in each of four pint-size jars, then top with cherries, almonds, and shredded coconut.

Enjoy them warm or store them in the refrigerator for up to 4 days.

Nutritional Information (385 g per serving)

- Calories 745

- Fats 55 g
- Carbs 58 g
- Protein 16 g
- Sodium 76 mg

Pancakes with Quinoa and Blueberries

Servings: 4

Ingredients

¾ cup all-purpose flour 1 cup cooked quinoa

2 tbsp. baking powder

½ teaspoon of salt

1 big egg

1 big egg white

¼ cup low-fat milk 1 tablespoon unsalted butter, melted

2 tbsp of maple syrup

½ cup fresh blueberries

Nonstock cooking spray

Preparation

1. In a medium mixing basin, combine the quinoa, flour, baking powder, and salt.

2. Combine the egg, egg white, melted butter, and maple syrup in a separate basin.

3. Mix the wet and dry ingredients. Stir to ensure that everything is well integrated. Incorporate the blueberries into the batter.

4. Melt butter in a non-stick pan or griddle over medium-high heat. Coat it with non-stick frying spray and scoop the batter into it in spoonful. When bubbles appear in the batter, turn the pancakes and cook for another 2 minutes on the other side.

5. Continue until all of the batters have been utilized.

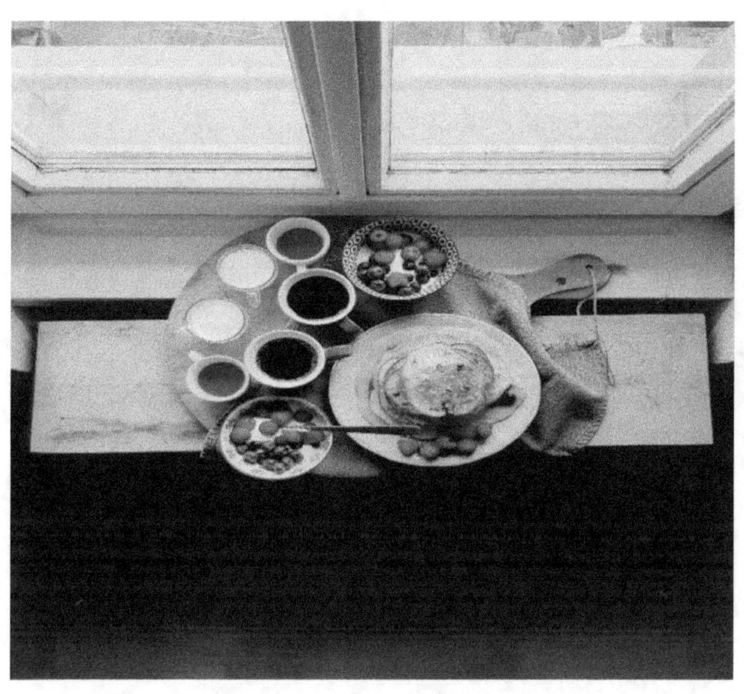

Nutritional Information (138 g per serving)

- Calories 233
- Fats 6 g
- Carbs 38 g
- Protein 8 g
- Sodium 45 mg

Ingredients for Cinnamon Apple Quinoa Parfait

Servings: 4

1 pound rolled oats

1 ½ teaspoons melted coconut oil

2 tsp. granulated sugar

2 tablespoons cinnamon powder, divided

four apples

a tsp vanilla extract

1 teaspoon of brown sugar

1 cup of water

3 cups quinoa, cooked

2 cups vanilla non-fat Greek yogurt

Preparation

1. Preheat the oven to 350 degrees Fahrenheit. Use parchment paper to line a 13x9 baking pan.

2. Combine the oats, coconut oil, granulated sugar, and 1 teaspoon of cinnamon in a small mixing basin. Spread the oat crumble on the prepared baking sheet and bake for 10 minutes or until golden brown. Set it aside and let it cool.

3. Core and peel the apples. Chop them roughly into pieces.

4. Combine the apple pieces, 1 teaspoon cinnamon, vanilla, brown sugar, and water in a medium saucepan. Bring the water to a boil over medium heat, then lower it to low heat and continue to cook until the apples are tender and have a syrupy consistency. Allow it to cool fully before refrigerating it for an hour.

5. Layer the yogurt, quinoa, and apple compote in four glasses, in that sequence. Repeat these layers two more times, finishing with the oat crumble.

Nutritional Information (433 g per serving)

- Calories 417
- Fats 10 g
- Carbs 67 g
- Protein 17 g
- Sodium 52 mg

Muffins with Avocado Quinoa Frittata

Servings: 12

Ingredients

1 quinoa cup

2 cup water

3 huge eggs

3 huge egg whites

1 cup chopped spinach

2 teaspoons chopped cilantro

¼ cup chopped red onion 1 small red bell pepper, diced

1 chopped ripe avocado

½ cup shredded mozzarella, salted and peppered to taste

Preparation

1. Bring the quinoa and water to a boil in a small saucepan over high heat.

Reduce the heat to low and cook for 15 minutes, or until all of the liquid has been absorbed. Cover with a lid and let aside for 10 minutes. Using a fork, fluff the rice. Set it aside and let it cool.

2. Preheat the oven to 350 degrees Fahrenheit. Line a 12-cup muffin pan with muffin liners.

3. In a medium mixing bowl, combine the eggs and egg whites. Combine the spinach, cilantro, bell pepper, onion, avocado, salt, pepper, cheese, and quinoa in a mixing bowl.

4. Divide the mixture equally among the muffin cups. Bake the eggs for 20-25 minutes, or until they are set.

5. Allow the frittatas to cool for at least 5 minutes on a wire rack before serving, or keep them in the fridge for up to 7 days.

Nutritional Information (69 g per serving)

- Calories 119
- Fats 6 g
- Carbs 12 g
- Protein 6 g
- Sodium 65 mg

Recipes for Soup, Salad, and Bowls

Black Bean, Sweet Potato Quinoa Chili

Servings: 4

Ingredients

1 tbsp olive oil

1 chopped onion

5 garlic cloves, chopped

1 ½ teaspoon chili powder

1 tablespoon coriander powder

1 can (14 oz.) roasted tomatoes

½ pound washed dry black beans

1 chipotle Chile, minced (from a can of chilies in adobo sauce)

1 teaspoon dried oregano

5 cup water

2 tsp sea salt

1 ½ cups diced sweet potatoes

¼ cup quinoa

Sour cream, green onions, and cilantro are optional garnishes.

Preparation

1. Heat the oil in a large skillet over medium heat. Fry the onion for 6 minutes, or until it becomes golden. Cook for approximately a minute after adding the garlic, chili powder, and coriander.

2. Bring the can of tomatoes, beans, chipotle pepper, oregano, and water to a boil in a saucepan. Reduce to low heat and cover with a lid. Allow for a 12-hour simmer.

3. Stir in the sweet potatoes and quinoa, and cook until the beans are mushy and the sweet potatoes are tender. If the chili gets too thick, add additional water to thin it down.

4. Season with salt and pepper immediately before serving.

Warm with sour cream, green onions, and cilantro is best.

Nutritional Information (527 g per serving)

- Calories 290
- Fats 2 g
- Carbs 56 g
- Protein 15 g
- Sodium 86 mg

Ingredients for Quinoa Vegetable Soup

Servings: 6

3 tablespoon olive oil

1 chopped onion 3-4 minced garlic cloves

2 peeled and sliced carrots

1 zucchini, chopped 2 celery stalks

1 tiny chopped red bell pepper

1 diced sweet potato

To taste, season with salt and freshly ground black pepper.

½ teaspoon dried thyme

1 teaspoon dried basil

one bay leaf

1 teaspoon red pepper flakes, to taste

1 can chopped tomatoes (28 oz.)

1 cup washed quinoa

6 cups chicken or veggie stock

2 cup water

1 can (15 ounces) of washed and drained chickpeas

2 cups trimmed and sliced kale

1 tsp. lemon juice

If preferred, top with freshly grated Parmesan cheese.

Preparation

1. In a soup stockpot or Dutch oven, heat the oil over medium heat.

Cook for 1 minute, or until the onion and garlic cloves are aromatic.

Sauté the carrot, celery, zucchini, red bell pepper, and sweet potato for 5-7 minutes, or until soft.

Season with salt and pepper to taste. Take the pan off the heat.

2. Combine the thyme, basil, bay leaf, red pepper flakes, diced tomatoes, quinoa, stock, and water in a mixing bowl. Stir the items together a few times. Bring the water to a boil over high heat. Once boiling, remove the lid and decrease the heat to medium-low. Allow the soup to cook for 25 minutes before adding the chickpeas and greens. Simmer for another 5-8 minutes, or until the kale is soft.

3. Taste and adjust seasoning with salt and pepper as needed. Add the lemon juice. To blend, stir everything together. Take the pan off the heat.

4. Remove the bay leaf before serving. If preferred, top with grated parmesan.

Nutritional Facts (165 g per single serving)

- Calories 280
- Fats 10 g
- Carbs 32 g
- Protein 12 g
- Sodium 1920 mg

Soup with Quinoa, White Beans, and Kale in the Slow Cooker

Servings: 6

Ingredients

¾ cup rinsed quinoa

split 4 cups of chicken broth

1 teaspoon minced garlic

½ cup chopped yellow onion

two teaspoons of Seasoning from Italy

Season with salt and pepper to taste.

1 can chopped tomatoes (14 oz.)

2 cannellini beans (15 ounces)

3 cups kale, chopped

Preparation

1. Combine the rinsed quinoa, 2 cups broth, garlic, onion, Italian seasoning, salt, and pepper in a slow

cooker. Stir in 1 can of cannellini beans and 1 can of canned tomato (with liquids).

2. Combine the remaining broth and cannellini beans in a food processor. Pour the ingredients into the slow cooker and stir well. Cook on high for 3-4 hours or low for 5-6 hours, covered.

3. Prepare the greens around 20 minutes before serving. Remove the stems and wash them before chopping them into bite-sized pieces.

4. Taste and adjust the soup's spices. Cook for another 15 minutes after adding the greens.

5. Serve right away.

Nutritional Information (143 g per serving)

- Calories 293
- Fats 2 g
- Carbs 53 g
- Protein 17 g
- Sodium 1219 mg

Salad with Grilled Halloumi and Quinoa

Servings: 2

Ingredients

½ cup washed quinoa

1 cup of water

2 tablespoons extra virgin olive oil

2 tablespoons fresh lemon juice

8 oz. halloumi (cut into 8 pieces)

½ lemon

3 cups lettuce and arugula leaves

¼ cup chopped flat-leaf parsley

2 teaspoons chopped mint

Cucumber pickled:

2 teaspoons red wine vinegar

½ teaspoon of sugar

1 garlic clove, chopped

⅛ teaspoon red pepper flakes

Season with salt and pepper to taste.

½ peeled and sliced cucumber

1 sliced scallion

Preparation

1. In a small saucepan, bring the quinoa and water to a boil over high heat. Reduce the heat to low and cook for 15 minutes, or until all of the liquid has been absorbed. Cover with a lid and let aside for 10 minutes. Toss the quinoa with olive oil and 2 tablespoons of lemon juice. Allow it to cool.

2. Preheat a grill pan or skillet to medium heat. Cook the halloumi slices till golden brown. Squeeze some lemon juice on top of the cheese.

3. To prepare the pickled cucumber, follow these steps: In a medium mixing bowl, combine the red wine vinegar, sugar, garlic, red pepper flakes, salt, and pepper. Combine the cucumber and scallions in a mixing bowl.

Set it aside for now.

4. Divide the quinoa between two clean plates. Serve with cucumber pickles, salad leaves, mint, parsley, and halloumi.

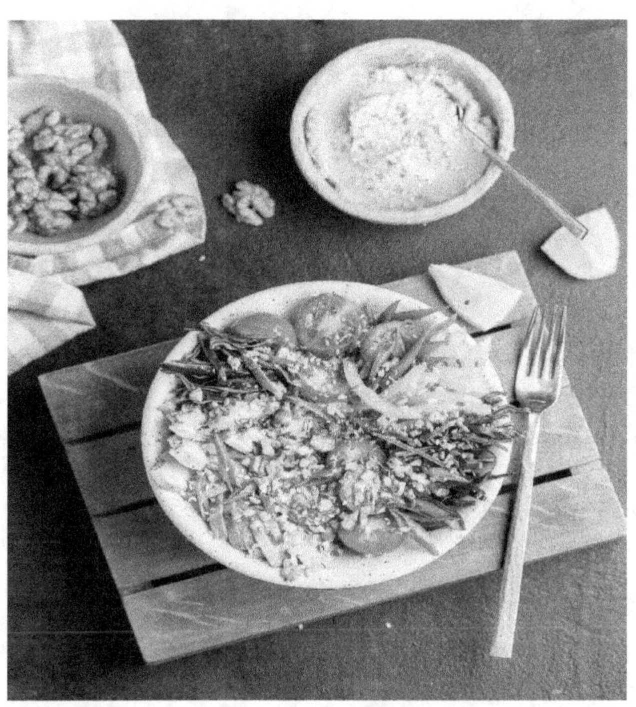

Nutritional Information (299 g per serving)

- Calories 664
- Fats 44 g
- Carbs 33 g
- Protein 33 g
- Sodium 24 mg

Salad of Sweet Potato Quinoa with Goat Cheese and Cherries

Servings: 4

Ingredients

1 cup quinoa, uncooked

1 cup of water

2 medium sweet potatoes (1-inch chunks)

½ teaspoon olive oil

¼ tsp garlic powder

⅛ teaspoon cumin

⅛ tsp cayenne pepper

⅛ teaspoon of salt

1 cup pitted and chopped luscious dark red cherries

¼ cup crumbled goat cheese

¼ cup walnuts toasted

Dressing:

1 ½ teaspoon olive oil for dressing

1 small lemon, squeezed

⅛ teaspoon cumin

1 minced garlic clove

1 tablespoon honey

Preparation

1. Bring the quinoa and water to a boil in a small saucepan over high heat. Reduce the heat to low and cook for 15 minutes, or until all of the liquid has been absorbed. Cover with a lid and let aside for 10 minutes. With a fork, fluff the quinoa. Place it aside to cool.

2. Preheat the oven to 400 degrees Fahrenheit. Using parchment paper, line a baking sheet.

3. Drizzle olive oil over the sweet potatoes, then season with garlic powder, cumin, cayenne pepper, and salt. Bake for 15 minutes, or until the potatoes are cooked.

4. In the meanwhile, make the dressing. Whisk together all of the dressing ingredients in a small bowl.

5. When the sweet potato is done, combine it with the quinoa in a large mixing dish. Pour the dressing over

the mixture and toss well. Combine the cherries, goat cheese, and walnuts in a mixing bowl.

Nutritional Information (185 g per serving)

- Calories 360
- Fats 14 g
- Carbs 50 g
- Protein 12 g
- Sodium 103 mg

Salad with Quinoa and Beans

Servings: 4

Ingredients

1 can (20 oz.) kidney beans, drained and rinsed

2 cups quinoa, cooked

1 finely sliced red onion

¼ cup feta cheese 1 cup basil, chopped

Dressing:

Juice from 2 lemons

½ cup virgin olive oil

2 tablespoon Dijon mustard

Season with salt and pepper to taste.

Preparation

1. In a small mixing bowl, combine the lemon juice, olive oil, and mustard to create the dressing. Season to taste with salt and pepper.

2. In a large mixing basin, combine the other ingredients EXCEPT for the cheese. Pour the dressing over the salad and toss to ensure that everything is completely covered.

3. Sprinkle the feta cheese over the salad.

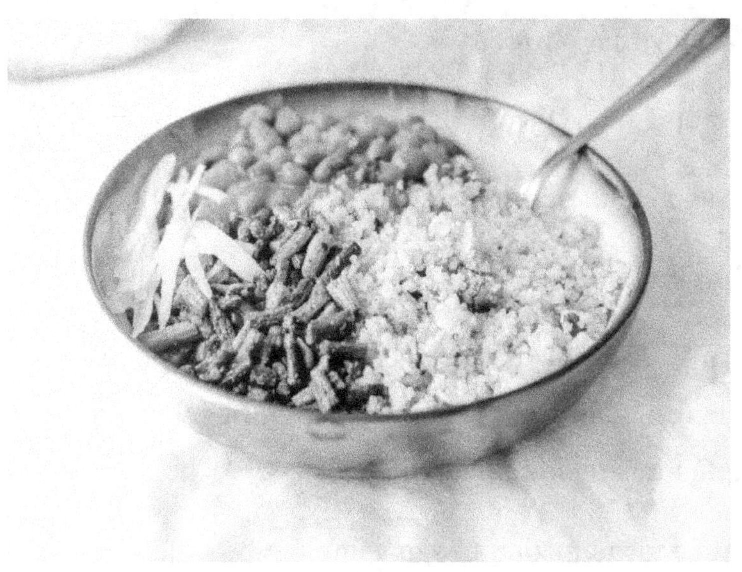

Nutritional Information (240 g per serving)

- Calories 471
- Fats 32 g
- Carbs 38 g
- Protein 11 g
- Sodium 276 mg

Quinoa Tabbouleh

Servings: 8

Ingredients

1 cup washed and drained quinoa

2 cup water

¼ cup virgin olive oil

2 tbsp of lemon juice

Season with salt and pepper to taste.

½ medium red onion, diced 2 medium tomatoes, minced 2 cups parsley, minced ½ cup mint, minced 2 garlic cloves, minced 8 ounces feta

Preparation

1. In a small saucepan, bring the quinoa and water to a boil over high heat. Reduce the heat to low and continue to simmer for 15 minutes, or until all of the liquid has been absorbed. Remove from the heat and set aside for 10 minutes. Using a fork, fluff the quinoa. Place the cooked quinoa in a large mixing dish to cool.

2. To create the dressing, mix the olive oil, lemon juice, and a sprinkle of salt in a small bowl.

3. Stir in the onions, tomatoes, parsley, mint, and garlic to the heated quinoa. Toss the salad with the

dressing to ensure that all of the components are uniformly covered.

4. Sprinkle the feta over the salad and serve right away.

Nutritional Information (111 g per serving)

- Calories 227
- Fats 14 g
- Carbs 18 g
- Protein 8 g
- Sodium 271 mg

Salad with Quinoa, Fennel, and Pomegranate

Servings: 8

Ingredients

1 cup washed quinoa

2 cup water

1 small lemon ¼ cup + 1 tablespoon olive oil

2 medium fennel bulbs, cut into 14-inch slices lengthwise

seasoned with salt & pepper

1 ½ teaspoons cumin powder

1 tablespoon sugar

1 seeded and chopped serrano chili

½ cup chopped fresh cilantro ½ cup chopped fresh mint

¼ cup pomegranate seeds 1 teaspoon minced fresh dill

Preparation

1. Bring the quinoa and water to a boil in a medium saucepan over high heat. Continue to simmer over low heat for approximately 15 minutes, or until all of the liquid has been absorbed. Remove from the heat and leave aside for 10 minutes, covered with a lid. Using a fork, fluff the rice.

Place the cooked quinoa in a large mixing basin.

2. Toss the quinoa with 1 tablespoon of oil and a couple of squeezes of lemon juice. Place aside.

3. Heat ¼ cup oil in a large pan over medium heat. Cook the fennel for approximately 10 minutes, or until soft. Season with salt & pepper and a splash of lemon juice. Cook for another minute after adding the cumin and sugar.

4. Combine the quinoa, fennel, herbs, and chili in a mixing bowl. Mix everything up well.

5. To serve, top the salad with a liberal sprinkling of pomegranate seeds.

Nutritional Information (101 g per serving)

- Calories 179
- Fats 10 g
- Carbs 20 g
- Protein 4 g
- Sodium 32 mg

Salad with Thai Quinoa and Peanut Dressing

Servings: 2

Ingredients

Thai peanut sauce:

2 tablespoons of peanut butter

1 teaspoon of soy sauce

1 tsp honey (or agave syrup)

½ jar of lime juice

½ teaspoon sesame oil

1 minced garlic clove

1 teaspoon grated fresh ginger

1 teaspoon chili flakes, or to taste

If necessary, thin it with water.

Salad

2 cups quinoa, cooked

1 small chopped red bell pepper 1 to 1 ½ cups shredded red cabbage

1 shredded carrot

2 tbsp. red onion, diced

½ cup cooked frozen shelled edamame ¼ cup raw cashew

2 finely sliced green onions

1-2 teaspoons chopped fresh cilantro

Preparation

1. Whisk together all of the dressing ingredients until smooth.

If required, add more water to get the desired consistency.

2. In a large mixing bowl, combine the quinoa, bell pepper, red cabbage, carrot, onion, edamame, cashews, green onions, and cilantro.

3. Toss the salad with the dressing to coat it.

Nutritional Information (515 g per serving)

- Calories 394
- Fats 7 g
- Carbs 69 g
- Protein 17 g
- Sodium 729 mg

Mediterranean Quinoa Bowl with Roasted Red Pepper Sauce

Servings: 1

Ingredients

½ cup cooked quinoa 2 tbsp olive oil

1 teaspoon of lemon juice

2 tablespoons chopped flat-leaf parsley

Season with salt and pepper to taste.

½ cup spinach

2 teaspoons feta cheese

kalamata olives, 2 tablespoons

2 tablespoon bell pepperoncini

1 tablespoon red onion, thinly sliced

hummus (two tablespoons)

roasted red pepper sauce 2 tablespoon

Preparation

1. Toss the quinoa with olive oil, lemon juice, and parsley in a medium mixing basin. Season to taste with salt and pepper.

2. Place the other ingredients on top of the quinoa.

3. Serve right away.

Nutritional Information (289 g per serving)

- Calories 484
- Fats 37 g
- Carbs 30 g
- Protein 10 g
- Sodium 451 mg

Broccoli Kale Quinoa Bowl

Servings: 6

Ingredients

1 medium broccoli floret, cut

2 cups shelled frozen edamame

4 cups kale, chopped

6 cups quinoa, cooked

1 peeled, pitted, and sliced avocado

½ cup sliced almonds

For garnish, toast sesame seeds

Vinaigrette with sesame and soy sauce

a third of a cup of vegetable oil

¼ tablespoon rice wine vinegar

1 teaspoon honey

2 tablespoon soy sauce

¼ teaspoon sesame oil

a pinch of black pepper and salt

Preparation

1. Steam the broccoli florets for 4-5 minutes, or until crisp and tender. Place them in a clean basin.

2. Place the frozen edamame in the steamer and heat for 5 minutes. Remove it from the pan and put it aside with the broccoli.

3. Whisk together all of the vinaigrette ingredients in a small bowl until thoroughly mixed.

4. Toss the kale with 2 tablespoons of the vinaigrette in a large mixing basin. Allow the kale to soften for 2 minutes after massaging it with the vinaigrette.

5. Divide the quinoa into four dishes. Add broccoli, kale, edamame, avocado, and nut slices on top. Drizzle the vinaigrette over the top and decorate with sesame seeds.

Nutritional Information (304 g per serving)

- Calories 393
- Fats 16 g
- Carbs 50 g
- Protein 18 g
- Sodium 28 mg

Recipes for Sandwiches, Bites, and Fritters

Quesadillas with Broccoli and Quinoa

Servings: 4

Ingredients

¼ cup quinoa, cooked

½ cup broccoli, chopped

1 cup cheddar cheese, shredded

Season with salt and pepper to taste.

4 whole-wheat tortillas, medium

2 tablespoon olive oil

Preparation

1. Combine the quinoa, broccoli, and cheese in a medium mixing basin. Season to taste with salt and pepper. Divide the mixture evenly across four tortillas, putting it just on one side of each tortilla so it can be folded over.

2. In a medium pan over medium heat, heat the oil. Cook two quesadillas in the pan for approximately 3 minutes on each side, or until golden and crispy. Repeat until all of the quesadillas are done.

3. Make wedges out of the quesadilla. Serve right away.

Nutritional Information (95 g per serving)

- Calories 279
- Fats 16 g
- Carbs 23 g
- Protein 11 g
- Sodium 399 mg

Crispy Quinoa Burger with Caramelized Beer Onions

Servings: 4

Ingredients

2 cups red quinoa, cooked

1 cup mashed cannellini beans

½ cup bread crumbs (panko)

1 big gently beaten egg

1 garlic clove, grated

1 teaspoon chili powder chipotle

½ teaspoon of salt

½ teaspoon black pepper

¾ cup shredded strong cheddar cheese

1 tablespoon melted butter

2 big finely sliced sweet onions

1 cup beer

1 tablespoon extra virgin olive oil

4 burger buns

4 eggs

4 slices Swiss cheese, such as Gruyere

Preparation

1. Combine the quinoa, cannellini beans, bread crumbs, 1 egg, grated garlic, chili powder, salt, and pepper in a medium mixing bowl. Stir in the shredded cheese well. Form the ingredients into four equal burger patties using somewhat moist palms. Place them on a clean dish and place them in the fridge for approximately 15 minutes to firm up.

2. Prepare the onions when you're ready to cook. Melt the butter in a large pan over medium–high heat. Cook for approximately 15 minutes after adding the onions. Pour the beer into three or four batches, allowing it to gently seep into the onions. Cook the onions until the beer has completely evaporated. Place the onions in a clean basin.

3. Heat a tablespoon of olive oil in the same skillet over medium heat. Cook for 5 minutes on each side, or until the patties are golden and crispy. In the final

few minutes of cooking, add the gruyere cheese and cover the pan with a lid. Cook until the cheese melts.

4. Meanwhile, cook the eggs to desired doneness in a small pan.

5. To assemble, put a thick layer of caramelized onions on each bun and top with a burger and an egg. Enjoy!

Nutritional Information (543 g per serving)

- Calories 743
- Fats 32 g
- Carbs 80 g
- Protein 30 g
- Sodium 1080 mg

Vegetable-stuffed Ingredients for Quinoa Burrito

Servings: 4

Ingredients

2 ½ tbsp olive oil, split

1 chopped onion

1 jalapeño, seeded and chopped ½ cup rinsed quinoa

4 minced garlic cloves

⅔ cup vegetable broth

1 cup thawed frozen corn

¾ cup grated zucchini

¾ cup diced tomatoes

⅓ cup plain Greek yogurt

1 tablespoon chopped fresh cilantro

2 tbsp. lime juice

1 tsp chipotle chili powder

4 whole grain tortillas

1 cup cheddar cheese, shredded

Preparation

1. Heat 1 tablespoon olive oil in a large pan over medium heat. Fry the onion and jalapeño until soft and tender, approximately 5–8 minutes. For 2 minutes, sauté the quinoa and garlic. Bring the broth to a boil in the saucepan.

2. Reduce the heat to low and cover the pan. Allow to simmer for 30-35 minutes, or until the majority of the liquid has been absorbed. Remove from the heat and let aside, covered, for 5-10 minutes.

Place in a clean basin.

3. Heat another tablespoon of olive oil in the same pan over medium-high heat. Cook for 2 minutes with the corn and zucchini.

Stir in the tomatoes and heat for another minute.

Put the veggies in a clean basin. With a paper towel, clean the skillet.

4. Combine the yogurt, cilantro, lime juice, and chili powder in a mixing bowl.

5. To build the tortilla, start with a layer of yogurt, then cheese, quinoa, and veggies. Roll it up and repeat to create three more wraps.

6. Heat 12 tbsp olive oil in a medium saucepan over medium heat. Place the burritos in the pan, seam side down, and cook until the tortillas are slightly brown on both sides.

Nutritional Information (274 g per serving)

- Calories 405
- Fats 15 g
- Carbs 18 g
- Protein 52 g
- Sodium 672 mg

Quinoa with Feta Zucchini Fritters

Servings: 10 fritters

Ingredients

½ cup quinoa

1 ½ cups water

2 grated zucchinis

3 eggs

5 tablespoons feta crumble

2 teaspoons chopped fresh dill

3 tablespoons olive oil, salted to taste

1 cup plain yogurt (served)

Preparation

1. Heat the quinoa and water in a medium saucepan over high heat. Bring the water to a boil, then lower it to low heat.

Continue to simmer for approximately 15 minutes, or until all of the liquid has been absorbed. Cover with a cover and set aside for 10 minutes to steam. Use a fork to fluff the quinoa. Place it in a medium bowl and set aside to cool fully.

2. Place the shredded zucchini in a sieve and season with a touch of salt. Allow it to rest in the sink for 10 minutes. Give it a brisk squeeze to get rid of any extra moisture.

3. Whisk the eggs in a separate dish. To make a batter, combine the feta, zucchini, dill, cooled quinoa, and a touch of salt.

4. Heat the oil in a large skillet over medium heat. One spoonful of the batter should be placed in the pan and gently pressed down with the back of a spatula. After around 5 minutes, flip the fritters once they are golden brown on one side. Fry the opposite side for another 4–5 minutes.

5. Serve immediately with a dollop of yogurt on the side.

Nutritional Information (86 g per serving)

- Calories 188
- Fats 8 g
- Carbs 8 g
- Protein 5 g
- Sodium 88 mg

Pico de Gallo Quinoa Nachos

Servings: 2

Ingredients

½ cup cooked quinoa

1 cup of water

½ cup shelled frozen edamame

½ cup thawed frozen corn

½ chopped red bell pepper

Tortilla chips, as much as you want (I used 2 ounces)

1 cup shredded reduced-fat mozzarella

Pico de gallo (pico de gallo):

2 diced tomatoes

1 tablespoon red onion, finely chopped

¼ fresh jalapeño, freshly chopped 1 sprig cilantro, finely chopped

1 tbsp olive oil (extra virgin)

1 lime, squeezed

Preparation

1. Preheat the oven to 375 degrees Fahrenheit.

2. Bring the quinoa and water to a boil in a small saucepan over medium-high heat. Reduce the heat to low and continue to cook for another 15 minutes, or until all of the liquid has been absorbed. Cover the quinoa for 10 minutes after adding the frozen edamame and corn.

3. Place the quinoa mixture in a large mixing basin. Add the chopped pepper and mix well.

4. In a small bowl, mix the tomatoes, onion, cilantro, and jalapeño to form the pico de gallo. Toss with olive oil and lime juice.

5. Arrange a layer of tortilla chips in an oven-safe pie dish, followed by the quinoa mixture, pico de gallo, and ½ cup of mozzarella. Repeat the layers once more, finishing with the remaining cheese.

6. Bake for 10 minutes, or until the cheese is golden brown and bubbling. Serve immediately, garnished with more cilantro.

Nutritional Information (320 g per serving)

- Calories 399
- Fats 13 g
- Carbs 61 g
- Protein 14 g
- Sodium 160 mg

Sushi with Quinoa and Miso Dipping Sauce

3 rolls are made using the following ingredients:

1 cup well-rinsed quinoa

1 ½ cups water

½ cup white vinegar

2 tablespoons honey

2 tsp sea salt

3 sheets of Japanese nori seaweed

1 pitted, peeled, and sliced avocado

½ big peeled, seeded, and cut into matchsticks cucumber

1 medium peeled and grated beetroot

½ cups microgreens

To make the dipping sauce:

2 tablespoons miso white

1 teaspoon lime juice

2 tablespoons honey

1 teaspoon ginger, freshly grated

1 teaspoon sesame seeds

Preparation

1. Cook the quinoa and water in a medium saucepan
over high heat. Bring the water to a boil, then lower it
to low heat.

Continue to simmer for approximately 15 minutes, or
until all of the liquid has been absorbed.

2. Meanwhile, in a small saucepan over medium heat,
combine the rice vinegar, honey, and salt.

3. Mix the vinegar with the cooked quinoa. Toss the
ingredients together in a medium pot and cover with
a lid.

Continue to cook the quinoa on low heat until all of
the liquid has been absorbed. Remove from heat and
let aside to cool fully.

4. Once the quinoa has cooled, begin assembling the
sushi.

Layer a bamboo mat on top of a seaweed sheet on
the countertop.

5. Spread a third of the quinoa evenly over the
seaweed sheet, leaving a border around the borders.
Place the avocado, cucumber, beetroot, and
microgreens in the centre of the baking sheet.

6. Using the bamboo mat as a support, roll the seaweed sheet away from you. While rolling, give the sushi roll a thorough squeeze to ensure that it is tight. Dab a finger in water and moisten the ends of the seaweed sheet to seal the roll. Slice the roll into 6-8 pieces.

7. In a small dish, combine all of the dipping sauce ingredients. Serve the sauce beside the sushi.

Nutritional Information (275 g per serving)

- Calories 394
- Fats 14 g
- Carbs 59 g
- Protein 13 g
- Sodium 2041 mg

Buffalo Quinoa Muffin Bites

Serving: 12

Ingredients

2 big eggs 1 cup cooked quinoa

¼ cup shredded carrot

¼ cup celery finely diced

3 tablespoons buffalo wing sauce

¼ cup cheddar cheese, shredded

non-stick cooking spray

Dip in blue cheese:

½ cup plain non-fat Greek yogurt

2 tablespoons crumbled blue cheese

Preparation

1. Preheat the oven to 350 degrees Fahrenheit. Coat a 12-cup mini muffin pan with non-stick cooking spray.

2. Combine the quinoa, eggs, carrot, celery, buffalo sauce, and cheddar cheese in a large mixing basin. Divide the batter equally among the muffin cups.

3. Bake for 30 minutes, or until the dough has set and the tops have become golden.

4. Place the muffins on a cooling rack to cool fully.

5. To prepare the dip, combine the yogurt and blue cheese until well combined.

6. Toss the dip with the muffin bits.

Nutritional Information (48 g per serving)

- Calories 66
- Fats 4 g
- Carbs 5 g
- Protein 4 g
- Sodium 230 mg

Recipes for Main Dishes

Casserole with Chicken, Broccoli, and Quinoa

Servings: 8

Ingredients

1 quinoa cup

2 cups water

1 head broccoli, florets removed and coarsely chopped

2 tablespoons olive oil (divided)

⅓ cup breadcrumbs, panko

3 finely cut chicken breasts

Season with salt and pepper to taste.

2 tbsp unsweetened butter

2 tbsp. all-purpose flour

2 cups of low-fat milk

1 ½ cups shredded cheddar cheese, sliced

⅓ cup plain Greek yogurt

Preparation

1. Preheat the oven to 350 degrees Fahrenheit.

2. Bring the quinoa and water to a boil in a large saucepan over high heat. Reduce the heat to low and continue to cook for 15 minutes, or until all of the liquid has been absorbed. Cover with a lid after adding the broccoli. Allow 10 minutes for the pot to sit.

3. Heat a tablespoon of olive oil in a large pan over medium heat. Toast the panko for 3 minutes, or until it becomes golden.

Place on a clean platter.

4. Heat the remaining tablespoon of olive oil. Season the chicken breast with salt and pepper and sauté over medium-high heat until fully done. Take them off the fire and put them aside. When the chicken has partially cooled, chop it into bite-sized pieces.

5. Melt the butter in the same skillet until it bubbles. Add the flour and continue to mix until it forms a paste. Pour in the milk gradually, stirring frequently, for 3-4 minutes, or until the lumps are gone and the liquid thickens. Mix in the quinoa, broccoli, chicken, 1 cup of cheese, yogurt, and salt and pepper to taste.

6. Spread the remaining cheese over the top of the mixture in a 13x9 baking dish.

7. Bake for 5 minutes, or until the cheese browns and the dish becomes bubbling.

8. For added crunch, top the casserole with the toasted panko.

Nutritional Information (269 g per serving)

- Calories 418
- Fats 19 g

- Carbs 25 g
- Protein 36 g
- Sodium 264 mg

Chicken Quinoa Parmesan Crispy

Servings: 4

Ingredients

1 quinoa cup

2 cups water

1 teaspoon of Italian seasoning

2 boneless, skinless chicken breasts, cut in half lengthwise

Season with salt and pepper to taste.

½ cup regular flour

2 big beaten eggs

½ cup shredded mozzarella

¼ cup Parmesan cheese, grated

1 cup tomato sauce

Preparation

1. Preheat the oven to 400 degrees Fahrenheit. Using parchment paper, line a baking sheet.

2. Bring the quinoa and water to a boil in a large saucepan over high heat.

Reduce the heat to low and continue to cook for 15 minutes, or until all of the liquid has been absorbed. Allow it to settle for 10 minutes before covering it with a lid. Fluff with a fork after adding the Italian spice. Put it away.

3. Season the chicken well with salt and pepper.

4. Separate the flour, eggs, and quinoa into three separate bowls.

5. Coat the chicken with flour, eggs, and quinoa. Press the quinoa into the meat to ensure it adheres.

6. Place the chicken on the prepared baking pan. Bake for 20-25 minutes, rotating halfway, or until golden brown.

Take the dish out of the oven.

7. Spoon marinara sauce over each piece of chicken, then top with the two slices of cheese. Bake for 5 minutes more, or until the cheese is completely melted and the chicken is cooked through.

8. For the finest crunch, serve immediately.

Nutritional Information (304 g per serving)

- Calories 514
- Fats 15 g
- Carbs 46 g
- Protein 47 g
- Sodium 319 mg

Stir-fry with chicken, edamame, and quinoa

Servings: 4

Ingredients

⅓ cup raw quinoa

⅓ cup of water

¼ cup creamy peanut butter

2 tbsp of soy sauce

½ teaspoon honey

1 teaspoon vinegar (red wine)

3 minced garlic cloves

1 tbsp sesame oil (divided)

1-pound boneless, skinless chicken breast, diced

Season with salt and pepper to taste.

3 cups florets broccoli

1 medium finely sliced red bell pepper

1 pound edamame

Garnishes are optional. roasted peanuts, cilantro, spicy sauce crushed

Preparation

1. Bring the quinoa and water to a boil in a large saucepan over high heat.

Reduce the heat to low and continue to cook for 15 minutes, or until all of the liquid has been absorbed. Allow it to settle for 10 minutes before covering it with a lid. Set aside the quinoa after fluffing it with a fork.

2. Combine the peanut butter, soy sauce, honey, vinegar, and garlic in a small bowl. Stir until completely smooth.

3. Season the chicken well with salt and pepper.

4. Heat ½ tablespoon sesame oil in a large pan over medium-high heat. Cook the chicken until it is thoroughly cooked through. Place the chicken on a clean dish.

5. Heat the remaining sesame oil in the same skillet. Stir-fry the broccoli, red pepper, and edamame for 6 minutes, or until crisp-tender. Season with salt and pepper to taste.

6. Return the chicken to the pan and drizzle with the peanut sauce. Toss the ingredients together to cover everything with the sauce.

7. Reduce the heat to low. Warm everything through by stirring in the quinoa.

8. Serve with peanuts, cilantro, or spicy sauce as a garnish. It is best served warm.

Nutritional Information (299 g per serving)

- Calories 411
- Fats 18 g
- Carbs 26 g
- Protein 39 g
- Sodium 695 mg

Salmon with Quinoa Cured

Servings: 4

Ingredients

1 pound fillet salmon

1 teaspoon sea salt

2 teaspoon sugar, divided

½ teaspoon Chile paste, split 1 cup's sake

2 minced garlic cloves

1 quinoa cup

2 cups water

1 tablespoon fresh parsley, chopped

½ cup red bell pepper, finely chopped ½ cup carrot, finely chopped ¼ cup onion, finely chopped 2 ½ tablespoons olive oil, split

Season with salt and pepper to taste.

Preparation

1. Rub 1 teaspoon salt and 1 teaspoon sugar into the fish fillet. Cover it with plastic wrap and place it on a clean platter.

Refrigerate it for at least 2 hours.

2. Take the salmon out of the refrigerator and rinse it under cold water to remove any extra salt and sugar. Dry the salmon with a paper towel.

3. In a transparent plastic bag, combine a cup of sake, 1 teaspoon of sugar, the Chile paste, and chopped garlic. To the mixture, add the salmon. Toss it to coat the fish well with the marinade. Refrigerate it for at least an hour.

4. Bring the quinoa and water to a boil in a large saucepan over high heat.

Reduce the heat to low and continue to cook for 15 minutes, or until all of the liquid has been absorbed. Allow it to settle for 10 minutes before covering it with a lid. Fluff the quinoa with a fork and sprinkle with the parsley. Put it away.

5. Heat 1 teaspoon of olive oil in a large pan over medium-high heat. for 2 minutes, or until the onion turns translucent, sauté the pepper, carrot, and onion. Toss the quinoa with the cooked veggies. Add ½ teaspoon olive oil and season with salt and pepper.

6. Heat another teaspoon of olive oil in the same skillet over medium-high heat. Fry the salmon for 5 minutes with the skin side down. Cover the pan with a cover to allow the salmon to finish cooking.

7. In the meanwhile, heat the marinade in a small saucepan. Bring everything to a boil over medium-high heat and simmer until the sauce is reduced to about ½ cup.

8. Turn the salmon skin-side up and pour the reduced marinade over it. Cook for another 5 minutes, or until well done.

9. Serve the fish with the quinoa right away.

Nutritional Information (206 g per serving)

- Calories 357
- Fats 12 g
- Carbs 33 g
- Protein 29 g
- Sodium 646 mg

Paella with Shrimp and Quinoa

Servings: 7

Ingredients

1 tablespoon extra virgin olive oil

1 chopped yellow onion 1 cored, seeded, and sliced red bell pepper

2 minced garlic cloves

1 ½ cups washed quinoa

3 cups chicken broth with a reduced salt content

¼ teaspoon red pepper flakes, crushed

one bay leaf

½ teaspoon paprika de Espana

½ teaspoon saffron threads, salt, and pepper to taste

½ cup sliced sundried tomatoes with olive oil

1 frozen cup of green peas

1 pound big peeled and deveined shrimp

Preparation

1. Heat the olive oil in a large pan over medium-low heat. Cook for approximately 5 minutes, or until the onions are transparent. Cook for another 5 minutes after adding the bell pepper. Fry for another minute after adding the garlic.

2. Combine the quinoa, chicken broth, red pepper flakes, bay leaf, paprika, salt, and black pepper in a mixing bowl. Scatter the saffron threads into the pan after rubbing them between your fingers. Bring the broth to a boil, covered. Reduce the heat to low and continue to cook for another 10-15 minutes, or until the majority of the liquid has been absorbed.

3. Add the sun-dried tomatoes, peas, and shrimp and mix well. Cook for another 5 minutes, covered. Remove from heat and let aside for 10 minutes.

4. Remove the bay leaf and serve while still heated.

Nutritional Information (236 g per serving)

- Calories 233
- Fats 5 g
- Carbs 28 g
- Protein 21 g
- Sodium 338 mg

Quinoa with Ground Beef from Mexico

Servings: 4

Ingredients

1 ½ tablespoon olive oil, split

12 oz. ground beef

2 minced garlic cloves

1 minced jalapeno

1 quinoa cup

1 cup veggie broth

1 (15 oz.) can of black beans, washed and drained

1 can chopped tomatoes (14 oz) (or use fresh)

1 cup kernels of corn

1 tsp. chili powder

½ tablespoon cumin

Season with salt and pepper to taste.

One lime juice

2 tbsp fresh cilantro leaves, chopped

1 seeded, peeled, and diced avocado

Preparation

1. Heat 12 tbsp olive oil in a large pan over medium-high heat. Stir-fry the ground beef until it is well done.

While cooking, split the ground beef into smaller pieces using the back of a spatula. Remove any extra fat from the cooked meat and place it in a clean dish.

2. Heat 1 tablespoon olive oil in the same skillet over medium-high heat. For approximately a minute, fry the garlic and jalapeño.

3. Combine the quinoa, vegetable broth, black beans, tomatoes, corn, chili powder, cumin, salt, and pepper in a mixing bowl. Bring the mixture to a boil, then lower to low heat and continue to simmer until the liquid has been entirely absorbed. Remove from heat, cover, and set aside for 10 minutes.

4. Combine the cooked ground beef, lime juice, and cilantro in a mixing bowl.

5. Garnish with avocado and serve right away.

Nutritional Information (431 g per serving)

- Calories 615
- Fats 33 g
- Carbs 57 g
- Protein 27 g
- Sodium 315 mg

Ingredients for Quinoa Beef Stew

Servings: 6

1 tablespoon extra virgin olive oil

2 pounds eye of round roast beef, cut into 1-inch cubes 1 big onion, finely chopped 4 large carrots, sliced

Season with salt and pepper to taste.

3 cups chicken broth with a reduced salt content

1 teaspoon corn-starch

8 chopped garlic cloves

three bay leaves

5 black peppercorns

1 cup washed quinoa

2 c. water

2 tsp garlic powder

1 frozen cup of peas

⅓ cup chopped parsley

Preparation

1. Heat the olive oil in a large pan over medium heat. 5 minutes, or until the onions are transparent, sauté the onions and carrots. Place in a clean basin.

2. Season the beef cubes with salt and pepper in the same skillet over medium-high heat until browned and cooked through.

3. Combine the corn-starch and chicken stock in a mixing bowl and pour over the meat. Combine the sautéed onion and carrots with the garlic, bay leaves, and peppercorns.

4. Bring to a boil, then cover and reduce to low heat. Continue to cook for 45 minutes.

5. Meanwhile, prepare the quinoa. Bring the quinoa and water to a boil in a large saucepan. Reduce the heat to low and continue to cook for another 15 minutes, or until most of the liquid has been absorbed. Remove from the heat and set aside for 10 minutes. With a fork, fluff the quinoa. Set aside while you wait for the meat to cook.

6. Remove the bay leaves and peppercorns after the meat is done.

7. Combine the garlic powder, quinoa, peas, and parsley in a mixing bowl. Serve warm.

Nutritional Information (391g per serving)

- Calories 370
- Fats 10 g
- Carbs 29 g
- Protein 43 g
- Sodium 421 mg

Quinoa Cake with Swiss Chard and Ham

Servings: 6

Ingredients

1 ¼ cup quinoa, uncooked

2 ½ cups water

5 tbsp extra-virgin olive oil (divided)

2 finely sliced onions

1 teaspoon thyme leaves, fresh

1 ½ pound Swiss chard, ribs removed, leaves ¼ pound sliced ham, finely chopped, cut into ¼-inch strips

Season with salt and pepper to taste.

1 cup grated Parmesan cheese 2 eggs

split ¾ cup panko breadcrumbs

Preparation

1. Bring the quinoa and water to a boil in a medium saucepan over high heat. Continue to simmer over low heat for approximately 15 minutes, or until all of the liquid has been absorbed. Remove from the heat and place a lid on top. Allow it to settle for 10 minutes. Fluff with a fork and place in a large mixing basin to chill.

2. Heat 3 tablespoons olive oil in a large pan over medium heat. Cook the onions and thyme for approximately 15 minutes, or until the onions are tender and golden brown.

3. Turn the heat up to medium-high. Season with salt and pepper and stir in the chard and ham. Cook for 5 minutes, or until the chard has wilted. Place it on a platter.

4. Stir in the Parmesan, eggs, ¼ cup panko, and salt and pepper to taste. Form the mixture into 12 3-inch-wide, ½-inch-thick patties.

5. Heat 2 tablespoons olive oil in a heavy-bottomed pan over medium heat.

6. Coat the patties with the remaining panko and cook in the pan, flipping halfway, until the breadcrumbs are golden brown and crispy.

7. To serve, top the patties with the ham and chard.

Nutritional Facts (146 g per single serving)

- Calories 409
- Fats 22 g
- Carbs 38 g
- Protein 18 g
- Sodium 628 mg

Lamb Chops with Spiced Quinoa and Lemon

Servings: 4

Ingredients

1 tablespoon cumin powder

¼ teaspoon chili flakes 1 garlic clove, minced

1 lemon juice

four tbsp olive oil

Season with salt and pepper to taste.

1 ½ cups washed quinoa

3 cups water

5 sliced spring onions

8 lamb loin chops

1 cup florets broccoli

Preparation

1. To create the marinade, combine the cumin, garlic, Chile, lemon juice, olive oil, salt, and pepper in a small bowl.

2. Toss the lamb chops with half of the marinade in a large mixing basin. Set aside both dishes.

3. Bring the quinoa and water to a boil in a large pot to prepare. Reduce the heat to low and continue to

cook for another 15 minutes, or until most of the liquid has been absorbed.

Take the pan off the heat and whisk in the remaining marinade.

Cover and put aside for 10 minutes. With a fork, fluff the quinoa and stir in the spring onion.

4. Melt butter in a griddle pan or skillet over high heat. Grill the lamb for 3–5 minutes on each side, or until done to preference.

5. Steam the broccoli till soft while the beef is cooking.

6. Plate the lamb with the quinoa and cooked broccoli.

Nutritional Information (362 g per serving)

- Calories 846
- Fats 51 g
- Carbs 45 g
- Protein 53 g
- Sodium 150 mg

Quinoa Fried Rice with Vegetables

Servings: 4

Ingredients

½ cup long-grained rice

½ cup cooked quinoa

2 cups water

3 tbsp olive oil (divided)

3 whisked eggs

1 finely diced tiny onion

1 finely chopped tiny carrot

½ cup coarsely chopped green bell pepper

½ cup chopped broccolini stems

2 tablespoons of soy sauce

3 minced garlic cloves

The spice of black pepper

1 cilantro sprig, finely chopped

2 tbsp sesame seeds, to taste

Preparation

1. Bring the rice, quinoa, and water to a boil in a large saucepan over high heat. Cover and reduce the heat to low. Simmer for 15 minutes, or until the majority of the liquid has been absorbed. Drain any extra water and put it aside to let the steam escape.
(Alternatively, use a rice cooker to cook the rice and quinoa.)

2. Heat 1 tablespoon oil in a large pan over medium heat.

Scramble the eggs until they are fully done. Place them on a clean platter.

3. Heat the remaining oil in the same skillet over medium-high heat. Cook the onion for 3–4 minutes, or until it is transparent.

For approximately 2 minutes, stir in the carrot and bell pepper. Cook for 2 minutes after adding the garlic and broccolini.

4. Toss the cooked rice and quinoa with the veggies, then season with soy sauce and pepper. Fry the rice until it is well heated.

5. Garnish with cilantro and sesame seeds and serve immediately.

Nutritional Information (274 g per serving)

- Calories 270
- Fats 5 g
- Carbs 44 g
- Protein 13 g
- Sodium 807 mg

Squash, tomato, and red pepper Ingredients for Quinoa Gratin

Servings: 6

3 tsp olive oil (divided)

2 cups red onion, chopped

1 ½ cups chopped red bell pepper

1 tablespoon minced garlic

1 pound yellow squash, sliced ¼-inch thick

½ cup quinoa, cooked

½ cup finely sliced fresh basil, divided ¾ teaspoon salt, divided

½ teaspoon black pepper ½ teaspoon fresh thyme

1 ½ oz baguette, roughly ripped

½ cup 2% milk with decreased fat

¾ cup shredded Gruyere cheese

3 big, gently beaten eggs

non-stick cooking spray

1 (12-ounce) beefsteak tomato, seeded and sliced

Preparation

1. Preheat the oven to 375 degrees Fahrenheit.

2. Heat 2 tablespoons of oil in a large pan over medium heat.

Cook until the onions are transparent, approximately 3-4 minutes. Cook for 2 minutes after adding the bell pepper and garlic. Cook for another 4 minutes after adding the squash. Place the cooked veggies in a large mixing basin. Toss the veggies with the quinoa, half the basil, ½ teaspoon salt, thyme, and pepper.

3. Pulse the baguette into coarse crumbs in a food processor.

4. In the same skillet, heat 1 teaspoon of oil over medium-high heat. For around 3 minutes, toast the bread crumbs. Place in a clean basin.

5. In a medium mixing basin, combine ¼ teaspoon salt, milk, cheese, and eggs. Combine the milk and vegetable mixtures in a mixing bowl. Place the mixture in an 11x7 baking dish.

6. Arrange the tomato slices on top of the veggie mixture. Sprinkle the toasted breadcrumbs over the top.

7. Bake for 40 minutes, or until golden brown on top.

8. Garnish with the remaining basil and serve right away.

Nutritional Information (375 g per serving)

- Calories 207
- Fats 8 g
- Carbs 23 g
- Protein 12 g
- Sodium 568 mg

Ingredients for Quinoa Stuffed Portobello Mushrooms

Servings: 4

⅓ cup washed quinoa

⅔ cup of water

4 big Portobello mushrooms, removed stems

1 tablespoon extra virgin olive oil

two tbsp balsamic vinegar

Season with salt and pepper to taste.

½ cup breadcrumbs 1 cup chopped tomatoes

¼ cup chopped fresh basil ½ cup fat-free feta cheese

¼ teaspoon red pepper flakes, crushed

Preparation

1. Preheat the oven to 375 degrees Fahrenheit.

2. Bring the quinoa and water to a boil in a medium saucepan over high heat. Reduce the heat to low and simmer for 15 minutes, or until most of the liquid has

been absorbed. Remove from the heat, cover, and put aside for 10 minutes to cool.

3. Arrange the mushrooms on a baking sheet, gill-side up. Brush them with oil and drizzle with balsamic vinegar. Season with salt and pepper to taste. 10 minutes in the oven.

4. Meanwhile, in a medium mixing bowl, combine the quinoa, tomatoes, breadcrumbs, basil, feta cheese, red pepper flakes, and salt and pepper to taste.

5. Take the mushrooms out of the oven and drain any extra liquid. Distribute the quinoa mixture among the mushrooms equally.

6. Bake for 12 minutes more, or until the cheese is melted.

Nutritional Information (187 g per serving)

- Calories 219
- Fats 9 g
- Carbs 26 g
- Protein 9 g
- Sodium 283 mg

Stuffed Bell Peppers with Quinoa in the Slow Cooker

Servings: 6

Ingredients

6 red bell peppers

1 cup washed quinoa

1 can (14 oz.) rinsed and drained black beans

1 can (14 oz.) of refried beans

1 ½ cup enchilada sauce red

1 tablespoon cumin

1 teaspoon chili powder

1 teaspoon onion powder

1 teaspoon salt

1 ½ cup mozzarella cheese, shredded

½ cup of water

Cilantro, avocado, and sour cream are optional garnishes.

Preparation

1. To prepare the bell peppers, do the following: Rinse the bell peppers well and wipe them dry with a paper towel. Remove the tops of the peppers and discard the ribs and seeds.

2. Combine the quinoa, beans, enchilada sauce, cumin, chili powder, onion powder, salt, and 1 cup of cheese in a large mixing basin. Fill the peppers with the quinoa mixture.

3. Fill a slow cooker with ½ cup water. Place the peppers in the slow cooker so that they are submerged in water. Cook on low for 6 hours or high for 3 hours, covered. Sprinkle the remaining ½ cup cheese on top of the peppers in the final 10 minutes of cooking. Cover and leave to melt the cheese.

4. Garnish with favourite toppings and serve immediately.

Nutritional Information (418 g per serving)

- Calories 379
- Fats 10 g
- Carbs 53 g
- Protein 20 g

- Sodium 901 mg

Desserts

Quinoa Cookies with Almonds and Cranberries

Servings: 24

Ingredients

1 ½ cups whole wheat white flour

1 teaspoon sea salt

½ teaspoon baking powder

½ teaspoon baking soda

1 unsalted butter stick, room temperature

¼ cup white sugar

¼ cup light brown sugar

¼ cup honey

2 huge eggs

a tsp vanilla extract

½ teaspoon almond extract

1 cup quinoa, cooked

1 pound rolled oats

1 cup cranberries, dried

½ cup sliced almonds

Preparation

1. Preheat the oven to 375 degrees Fahrenheit. Use parchment paper to line two 13x9 baking pans.

2. Combine the flour, salt, baking powder, and baking soda in a mixing bowl.

3. In a stand mixer, cream together the butter, sugar, light brown sugar, and honey until light and fluffy. Scrape the sides clean.

Add the eggs one at a time, ensuring that the first is well absorbed before adding the second. Pour in the vanilla and almond extracts.

4. Stir in the flour mixture in three batches until well-mixed.

5. Fold in the quinoa, oats, cranberries, and almonds using a spatula.

6. Spoon the batter onto the baking sheet with an ice cream scoop, leaving adequate space between the cookies.

7. Bake the cookies for 12 to 15 minutes, or until golden brown. Place them on a wire rack to cool fully.

Nutritional Information (47 g per serving)

- Calories 158
- Fats 6 g
- Carbs 24 g
- Protein 3 g
- Sodium 105 mg

Chocolate Quinoa Truffle

Servings: 24

Ingredients

⅓ cup quinoa

⅔ cup water

16 pitted whole dates

½ cup skin-on raw almonds

⅓ cup crunchy natural peanut butter

⅓ cup chocolate chips

Preparation

1. Bring the quinoa and water to a boil in a small saucepan over high heat. Reduce the heat to low and simmer for 15 minutes, or until all of the liquid has been absorbed. Allow it to settle for 10 minutes before covering it with a lid.

2. In the meanwhile, purée the dates in a food processor until they form a paste. Place the dates in a clean dish.

3. Place the almonds in a food processor. Pulse it a couple of times to coarsely cut them up.

4. In a food processor, combine the dates, peanut butter, and quinoa with the almonds. Pulse until all of the ingredients are mixed.

Add the chocolate chunks for one last pulse.

5. Make 24 balls out of the mixture. Refrigerate for at least one hour before serving to allow for firming.

Nutritional information (17 g per serving)

- Calories 80
- Fats 5 g
- Carbohydrates 8 g
- Protein 2 g
- Sodium 2 mg

Ingredients for Quinoa Brownies

Servings: 12

Ingredients

½ cup peeled and diced butternut squash

⅓ cup cocoa almond milk

3 teaspoons melted butter

1 tbsp maple syrup

⅔ cup of coconut sugar

1 cup quinoa, cooked

¼ cup oats rolled

½ cup whole grain flour

1 tsp. baking powder

two tbsp cocoa powder

4 tbsp ground flaxseed

1 cup chocolate chips, dark

non-stick cooking spray

Preparation

1. Preheat the oven to 375 degrees Fahrenheit. Use nonstock cooking spray to grease a 9x9 square baking pan.

2. Place the butternut squash in a microwave-safe dish and wrap it in plastic wrap. Cook for 4 minutes, or until the potatoes are fork-tender.

3. Puree the squash and almond milk together with an immersion blender or normal blender. Fill a large mixing bowl halfway with the mixture.

4. Stir in the butter, maple syrup, and sugar using a rubber spatula. Combine the quinoa, oats, flour, baking powder, cocoa powder, and powdered flax in a mixing bowl. Mix until everything is just blended. Mix in the chocolate chips.

5. Pour the mixture into the prepared baking dish. Bake for 25 minutes, or until a toothpick inserted into the centre comes out clean.

6. Allow the brownie to rest for at least 20 minutes before cutting into it.

Nutritional Information (74 g per serving)

- Calories 223
- Fats 11 g
- Carbs 29 g
- Protein 4 g
- Sodium 11 mg

Ingredients for Chocolate Quinoa Cake

Servings: 12

⅓ cup milk

4 eggs

a tsp vanilla extract

2 cups quinoa, cooked

¾ cup melted butter

½ cup granular sugar

1 cup cocoa powder, unsweetened

1 ½ tsp baking powder

½ tsp baking soda

½ teaspoon of sea salt

non-stick cooking spray

Frosting:

2 cups whipped heavy cream

1 cup chocolate chips, dark

Preparation

1. Preheat the oven to 350 degrees Fahrenheit. Line two circular cake pans with parchment paper and coat them with nonstock cooking spray.

2. Place the milk, eggs, and vanilla essence in a food processor and pulse a few times. Puree the quinoa and butter until the mixture is smooth, thick, and creamy.

3. Whisk together the sugar, cocoa powder, baking powder, baking soda, and salt in a large mixing basin.

4. Combine the wet and dry ingredients until fully blended.

5. Divide the batter evenly among the cake pans. Place the pans on the centre rack of the oven. 30 minutes in the oven, or until a toothpick inserted into the middle comes out clean. Take them out of the oven and leave them aside for 10 minutes. Place the cakes on a wire rack to cool fully, then peel off the parchment paper.

6. Meanwhile, boil the cream in a medium saucepan over medium heat until little bubbles form along the edges of the pan. In a medium glass dish, combine the chocolate chips.

To melt the chocolate, pour the hot cream over it. Stir until the mixture is smooth and shiny. Refrigerate the chocolate cream for at least 2-3 hours to allow it to cool fully.

7. Remove the chocolate cream from the refrigerator when ready to assemble. Whip the cream with an electric hand mixer until soft peaks form.

8. Place one of the cakes on a serving platter. Spread half of the whipped chocolate frosting on the cake layer, being careful not to go all the way to the edge. Place the next cake layer on top and cover with the remaining frosting.

9. Chill the cake in the refrigerator for 2-3 hours before serving.

Nutritional Information (101 g per serving)

- Calories 280
- Fats 15 g
- Carbs 36 g
- Protein 5 g
- Sodium 129 mg

Peanut Butter Quinoa Bar

Servings: 8

Ingredients

1 pound rolled oats

½ cup uncooked quinoa

1 cup of water

½ cup unsweetened peanut butter

¼ cup honey and ⅛ teaspoon salt

a tsp vanilla extract

1 teaspoon of coconut oil

¼ cup dark chocolate chips 1 tbsp chia seeds

Preparation

1. Preheat the oven to 350 degrees Fahrenheit. Line a 9-by-5-inch loaf pan with parchment paper.

2. Spread the quinoa and oats on a baking sheet. For 10 minutes, toast it in the oven.

3. Combine the oats and quinoa in a large mixing dish with the chia seeds.

4. Melt the peanut butter, salt, honey, vanilla extract, and coconut oil in a medium saucepan over low heat. Stir the mixture frequently until smooth and creamy.

5. Sprinkle the oats, quinoa, and chia seeds with the peanut butter mixture. Toss all of the ingredients together with a spatula to ensure that everything is

equally covered. Allow the mixture to cool for 5 minutes before adding the chocolate chips.

6. Pour the mixture into the prepared loaf pan and smooth it up with a spatula.

7. Freeze the pan for 10 to 20 minutes to firm it up.

8. Cut it into 8 bars and serve immediately or keep it in the fridge for later.

Nutritional Information (68 g per serving)

- Calories 312
- Fats 15 g
- Carbs 37 g
- Protein 9 g
- Sodium 5 mg

Ingredients for Salted Quinoa Fudge

Servings: 24

½ cup nut butter ½ cup protein powder

⅓ cup melted coconut oil

¼ tbsp cocoa powder

¼ cup pure maple syrup

1 medium banana, ripe

a tsp vanilla extract

1 teaspoon ground cinnamon

1 quinoa puffs cup

1 tsp flaky sea salt

non-stick cooking spray

Preparation

1. Blend the almond butter, protein powder, coconut oil, cocoa powder, maple syrup, banana, vanilla extract, and cinnamon in a food processor until smooth. Add the quinoa puffs and pulse a few times.

2. Divide the batter evenly between 24 silicone mini-muffin cups.

Sprinkle with salt.

3. Place the fudge in the freezer for approximately an hour to solidify.

Remove the fudge from the mold and serve immediately, or transfer it to a container to keep. They can be frozen for up to a month.

Nutritional Information (23 g per serving)

- Calories 97
- Fats 7 g
- Carbs 7 g
- Protein 3 g
- Sodium 108 mg

Coconut Milk Quinoa Pudding

Servings: 4

Ingredients

1 cup washed quinoa

4 cups coconut milk, unsweetened

⅓ cup pure maple syrup

1 ½ tsp vanilla extract

1 teaspoon ground cinnamon

¼ teaspoon of salt

Preparation

1. In a medium saucepan, combine all of the ingredients. Bring the water to a boil over medium heat. Reduce the heat to low and cover.

Allow boiling for 25 minutes, giving it a good toss every 5 minutes or so.

2. Remove the cover and simmer for another 5 minutes, or until the quinoa has absorbed most of the liquid.

3. Divide the quinoa pudding among four serving dishes. Allow 5-10 minutes for them to sit. The pudding will thicken more as it cools. Finish with a liberal sprinkling of cinnamon on top.

Nutritional Information (295 g per serving)

- Calories 670
- Fats 51 g
- Carbs 51 g
- Protein 11 g
- Sodium 180 mg

Bar with Quinoa and Chocolate Nuts

Servings: 18

Ingredients

2 tablespoons heated coconut oil 10 softened and pitted dates

1 cup nut butter

½ cup pumpkin seeds

1 quinoa puffs cup

½ cup coarsely chopped raw almonds

3 ½ ounces chopped 70% dark chocolate

⅓ cup shredded unsweetened coconut

Preparation

1. In a food processor, combine the dates and coconut oil to make a paste. Mix in the almond butter until all of the ingredients are combined. Place the mixture in a clean basin.

2. Gently fold in the pumpkin seeds, quinoa puffs, and almonds.

3. Line a baking sheet 8x10 with parchment paper. Spread the date mixture evenly on the tray, approximately ⅔ inches thick. Place it in the fridge to harden up.

4. In the meanwhile, melt the chocolate in a microwave-safe dish. Melt it on high for a minute, then remove it and mix it. If there are any lumps, return them to the microwave for 30 seconds at a time until the chocolate is smooth and shiny.

5. Evenly distribute the melted chocolate over the date mixture using a spatula. Sprinkle the shredded coconut on top of the chocolate.

Nutritional Information (48 g per serving)

- Calories 241
- Fats 17 g
- Carbs 20 g
- Protein 6 g
- Sodium 4 mg

Quinoa Crust Sweet Potato Pie

1 pie is made

Ingredients

1 cup cooked quinoa for the crust

½ cup regular flour

2 tbsp ground flaxseed

four tbsp maple syrup

4 tbsp. room temperature butter

non-stick cooking spray

Filling:

2 large sweet potatoes

A cup of almond milk

¾ cup brown sugar

1 teaspoon ground cinnamon

¼ teaspoon ground cloves ¼ teaspoon ground ginger

2 eggs

Preparation

1. Preheat the oven to 400 degrees Fahrenheit. Coat a pie plate with non-stick cooking spray.

2. Prepare the sweet potatoes by washing, peeling, and dicing them. Boil a kettle of water in a big saucepan. Cook for approximately 20 minutes, or until the sweet potatoes are fork soft. Drain the sweet potato and put it aside. Place the sweet potato in a microwave-safe bowl instead. Wrap in plastic wrap and microwave on high for 8-10 minutes.

3. Combine the quinoa, flour, flax, and maple syrup in a food processor. You want the crunchy parts in the quinoa, so don't overprocess it. Add the butter and pulse a few times to mix the ingredients.

4. Press the mixture into the prepared pie dish, ensuring sure the crust extends up the edges. 10 minutes in the oven.

5. In a clean food processor, combine the cooled sweet potatoes.

Blend in the almond milk until smooth. Blend in the sugar, spices, and eggs one more time.

6. Take the crust out of the oven. Fill the pie crust with the sweet potato mixture. Continue baking for another hour, or until a toothpick inserted into the

middle comes out clean. Cover with aluminium foil and continue baking if the top or crust is browning too rapidly.

7. Remove the pie from the oven and set aside for at least 30 minutes before serving.

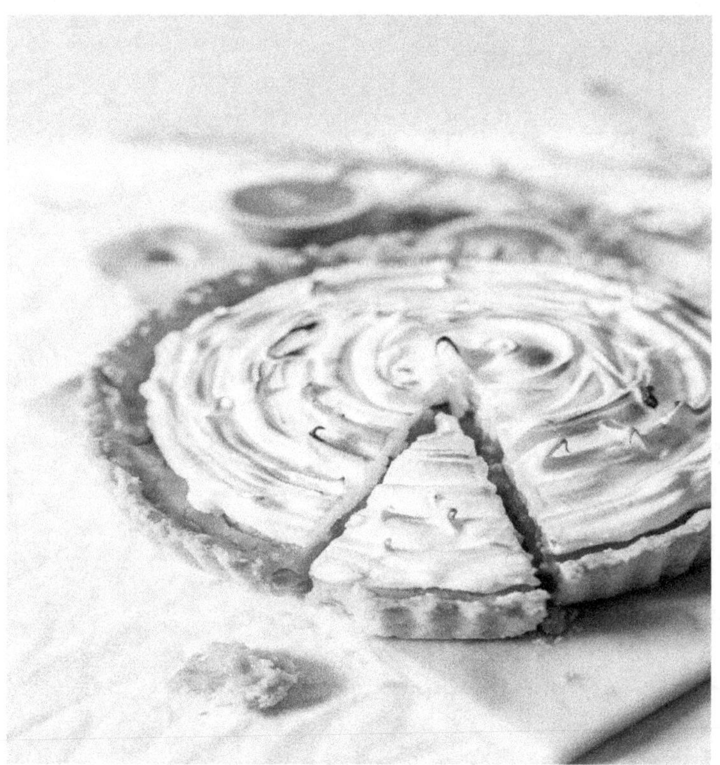

Nutritional Information (1130 g per pie)

- Calories 1959
- Fats 70 g

- Carbs 307 g
- Protein 36 g
- Sodium 535 mg

Chocolate Quinoa Bark

Servings: 24 pieces

Ingredients

½ cup pure maple syrup

2 tbsp of coconut oil

2 tsp. vanilla extract

2 tablespoons granulated instant coffee

1 tsp flaky sea salt

1 cup washed and dried quinoa

½ cup raw almonds, finely chopped

½ cup raw pecans chopped ¼ cup hemp seeds

¼ cup of chia seeds

½ fluid ounces chopped 90% dark chocolate

Cacao nibs and goji berries are optional toppings.

Preparation

1. Preheat the oven to 400 degrees Fahrenheit. Using parchment paper, line a baking sheet.

2. Melt the maple syrup and coconut oil in a large microwave-safe bowl for one minute on high. Combine the vanilla essence, instant coffee, and salt in a mixing bowl.

3. Mix the quinoa, almonds, and seeds with the liquid ingredients until everything is completely incorporated.

4. Evenly distribute the mixture on the baking sheet. Bake for 20-25 minutes, or until the quinoa has darkened and caramelized.

5. Melt the dark chocolate in a microwave-safe dish for one minute on high. Take it out of the microwave and give it a thorough stir. If there are any lumps, return them to the microwave for 30 seconds at a time until the mixture is smooth and shiny.

6. Spread the chocolate over the baking mixture until it forms a uniform layer. Garnish with cacao nibs and goji berries.

7. Place the chocolate bark in the refrigerator for at least 30 minutes to solidify. Remove the chocolate bark's parchment paper and cut it into 24 pieces.

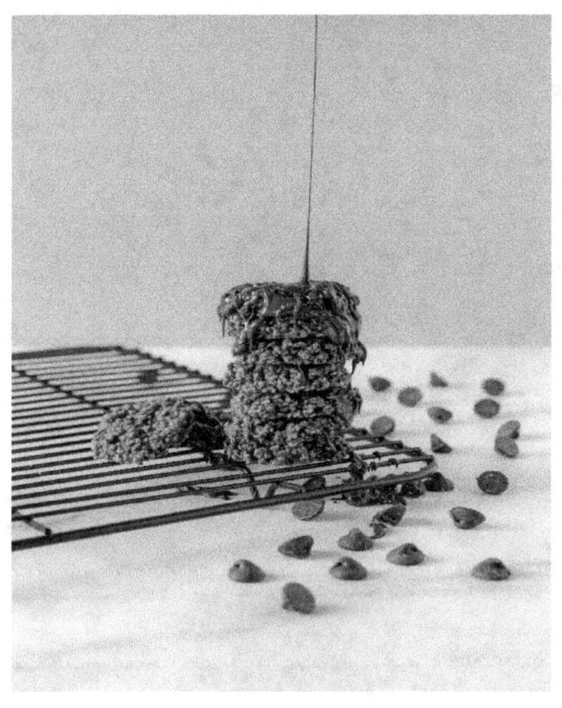

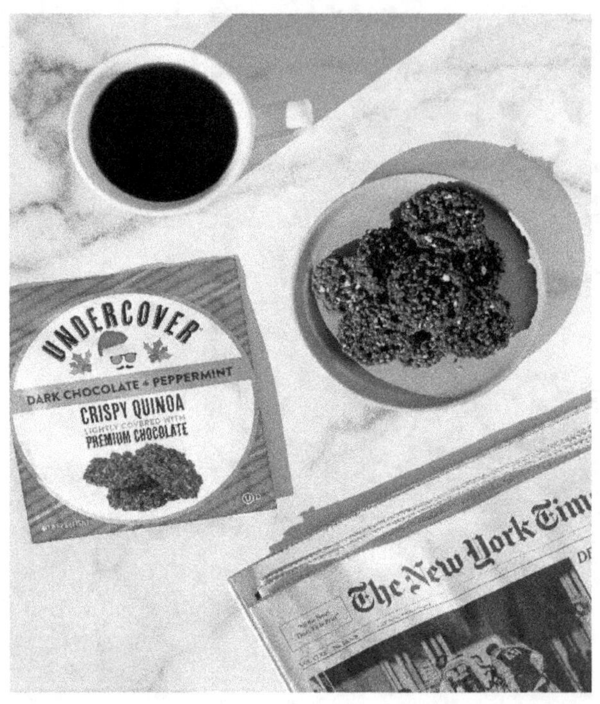

Nutritional Information (37 g per serving)

- Calories 181
- Fats 11 g
- Carbs 18 g
- Protein 4 g
- Sodium 11 mg

Honey olive quinoa cake

Servings: 1 cake

Ingredients

1 ½ cups whole grain flour

1 tsp. baking soda

1 tsp. baking powder

¼ teaspoon of salt

⅓ cup virgin olive oil

½ cup unprocessed honey

½ cup of buttermilk

two huge eggs

a tsp vanilla extract

12 cup almond flour

1 cup quinoa, cooked

¾ cup raisins

¼ cup unrefined honey

½ tsp almond extract

non-stick cooking spray

Preparation

1. Preheat the oven to 350 degrees Fahrenheit. Use non-stick cooking spray to grease an 8x8 square baking pan.

2. In a large mixing basin, combine the flour, baking soda, baking powder, and salt.

3. Combine the olive oil, honey, buttermilk, eggs, and vanilla essence in a separate dish.

4. Stir the wet ingredients into the dry ones with a rubber spatula until barely mixed. Fold in the ground almonds, quinoa, and raisins gently.

5. Pour the batter into the baking dish. Bake for 30–35 minutes, or until a toothpick inserted into the centre of the cake comes out clean. Take the dish out of the oven. Poke holes all over the cake using a toothpick.

6. Bring the honey and almond extract to a slow boil in a small saucepan. Drizzle the syrup slowly over the cake, allowing it to seep into the holes.

7. Allow the cake to cool for 10 minutes before serving.

Nutritional Information (989 g per cake)

- Calories 2804
- Fats 120 g
- Carbs 412 g
- Protein 63 g
- Sodium 890 mg

Crispy Quinoa Apple

Servings: 6

Ingredients

3 big peeled, cored, and thinly sliced apples

2 peeled, cored, and thinly sliced pears

Half a lemon juice

½ cup of coconut sugar

2 cups oats, rolled

¼ cup melted coconut oil 1 cup cooked quinoa

½ cup pure maple syrup

quinoa flour ½ cup

2 tablespoons ground cinnamon

non-stick cooking spray

Ice cream and maple syrup are optional garnishes.

Preparation

1. Preheat the oven to 350 degrees Fahrenheit. Non-stick cooking spray should be used to grease a pie pan.

2. Toss the pear and apple slices with the lemon juice and coconut sugar in a large mixing dish. Add the fruit to the pan.

3. In a separate mixing dish, combine the oats, cooked quinoa, coconut oil, and maple syrup. Stir in the quinoa flour until all of the ingredients are combined. Add the cinnamon and mix well.

4. Sprinkle the quinoa topping over the fruit. Bake for 35-45 minutes on the centre rack of the oven, or until the top begins to brown and the fruit begins to bubble. Cover with aluminium foil if the top is browning too soon.

5. Serve warm with ice cream and maple syrup on top.

Nutritional Information (268 g per serving)

- Calories 380
- Fats 11 g
- Carbs 72 g
- Protein 3 g
- Sodium 10 mg